YOUR KNOWLEDGE HAS VALUE

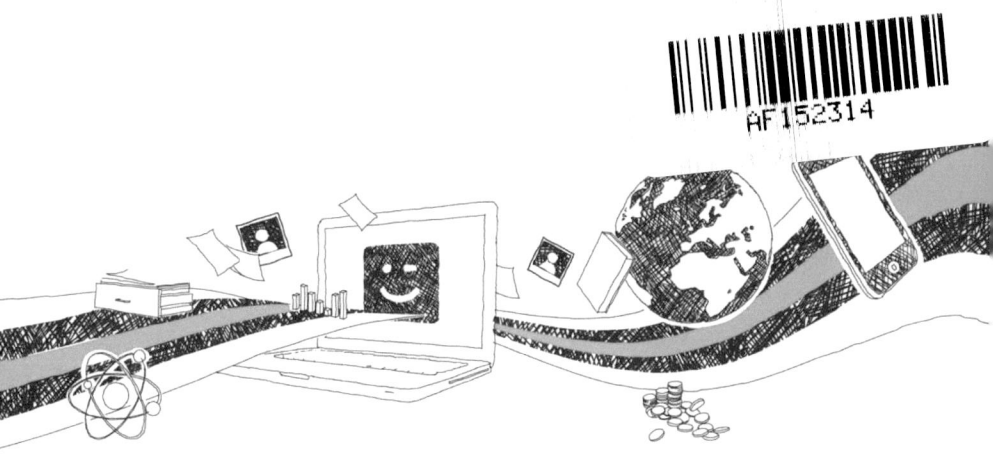

- We will publish your bachelor's and master's thesis, essays and papers

- Your own eBook and book - sold worldwide in all relevant shops

- Earn money with each sale

Upload your text at www.GRIN.com
and publish for free

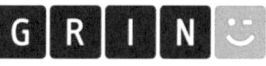

Carol Nganga

Attitudes Toward Hospice Care

GRIN Publishing

Bibliographic information published by the German National Library:

The German National Library lists this publication in the National Bibliography; detailed bibliographic data are available on the Internet at http://dnb.dnb.de .

Imprint:

Copyright © 2013 GRIN Verlag GmbH
Print and binding: Books on Demand GmbH, Norderstedt Germany
ISBN: 978-3-656-73944-9

This book at GRIN:

http://www.grin.com/en/e-book/280536/attitudes-toward-hospice-care

GRIN - Your knowledge has value

Since its foundation in 1998, GRIN has specialized in publishing academic texts by students, college teachers and other academics as e-book and printed book. The website www.grin.com is an ideal platform for presenting term papers, final papers, scientific essays, dissertations and specialist books.

Attitudes Toward Hospice Care

There is perhaps no more confusing mental process in life than attempting to define attitudes toward death. This process is even more complicated and impacting when it must be formulated by health practitioners who work in a hospice setting. It has been found that there exists a significant percentage (33%) of hospice nurses which found difficulty in knowing who controlled the overall responsibility of hospice patient care. Such confusion has led to an overwhelming desire by both community nurses and general practitioners for additional educational input from domiciliary services (Seamark, Thorne, Jones, Gray, & Searle, 1993, p. 57). There is little doubt that the health care professional finds themselves in a complex organizational system and must find a way to form their own outlook within that system. Nurses want to simultaneously maintain fidelity to patients and their family members, follow physician colleague orders, work in interdisciplinary family-centered teams, and yet follow their consciences when order care or treatments appear harmful to patients (Catlin et al., 2008, p. 106). The complexities of the situation in which hospice professionals find themselves in makes the defining of personal attitudes toward hospice care even more difficult.

There were an estimated 1.5 million patients who received hospice services in 2012 (NHPCO, 2013, p. 4). Therefore, a large patient population is directly effected by the outlooks which hospice clinicians take towards end of life care. Since the main focus of palliative care should be maximizing the quality of care of the hospice patient, health practitioners must adopt an attitude towards patients which maximizes the probability of the highest quality of life.

Normative Position

It is my personal belief that an ethically normative position towards dying patients and hospice which considers the input of patient and patients' families, along with a culturally empathetic outlook, should be adopted by health care professionals. Barrocas et al. (2010) defines normative ethics as "the branch of philosophical ethics concerned with formulating general standards or norms of ethical behavior and moral judgment." Health practitioners may find themselves in cases of hospice and end of life care where patients have to choose between respecting and obeying the wishes of the family of a dying patient or honoring the duty of patient by avoiding burdensome treatment which may produce detrimental harm through related complications (p. 676).

Normative ethics attempts to specify conditions which are non-ethical and determine when actions are correct. Such an example could include act-utilitarianism, which states that actions are only correct when they produce a minimum of an equal amount of happiness as would have been obtained from any other available alternative (Goldman, 1979, p. 90). This is why a normative outlook provides an excellent platform for hospice care providers as it considers crucial input from the patients themselves who are the only ones who actually know how they feel. Also, under a view of utility, one can provide a basis of recognizing true individual moral rights (Daniels, 2001, p. 316). Therefore, the considerations of the patient will be an utmost consideration in such ethical frameworks.

Patient Characteristic Considerations

The normative outlook also considers patient characteristics which may act as barriers to optimal patient health outcomes. One of the most effecting of such characteristics is the cultural/ethnic background of the patient. A culturally-sensitive approach is very applicable in a hospice care setting as there exist real and distinct cultural variations toward death and in the care of dying patients (Blair, 1995, p. 515).

The main goal of nursing is the aiding of individuals with the goal of attaining and maintaining an increases level of self-accord within their physical being, consciousness, and their spiritual essence (Barnett, 1991, p. 226). Therefore, it should be expected that variations in care outlooks will lead to alterations of patient input which will remain in line with their individual cultural perspectives. After all, it has been found that ethnicity influences common values and cultural beliefs which combine to influence end of life decision-making (Johnson, Kuchibhatla, & Tulsky, 2008, p. 1).

Ethnic characteristics of patients might also lead to barriers to hospice treatment in some circumstances. For example, it has been found that among African Americans there exist several barriers to hospice enrollment including misconceptions about hospice services, lacking of hospice service knowledge and awareness, preferences of more aggressive treatment, and deficits of trust in providers and the health system (Enguidanos, Kogan, Lorenz, & Taylor, 2011, p. 161).

Hospice clinicians should also consider additional characteristics of individuals so that they may tailor care plans accordingly. The presence of pain in older and minority hospice patients has been associated with race, physical function, gender, cognitive impairment, under treatment, and depression (Miller & Vince, 2002, p. 2). Even the sex of patients can have an impact on patient outcomes and treatment adherence as it has been found that women will entertain more positive attitudes toward the notion of hospice services than men due to long-long established observations that women tend to use health services more frequently as well as maintaining more positive attitudes toward them (Rainey, Crane, Breslow, & Ganz, 1984, p. 1999).

Communication Considerations

Healthy lines of communication between health care providers and their patients can result in positive health outcomes including improvement in life quality, well-being, and chances of survival (Levinson, Lesser, & Epstein, 2010, p. 1313). Therefore, an optimal outlook by clinicians on hospice care should include an emphasis of developing healthy lines of communication with their patients. Casarett et al. (2005) concluded that simple communication interventions are correlated with improvements in end-of-life care and decreases in the utilization of resources by promoting early and timely access to hospice resources in nursing home settings (p. 216).

Hospice clinicians must additionally be prepared to encounter angry communication within clinical environments. A normative outlook is also applicable here because when physicians empathize and engage with angry hospice patients there is a noted improvement in the patient's pain response as well as a reduction in patient suffering (Houston, 1999, p. 5). Such situations should once again remind physicians why a normative outlook should be applied toward lines of patient-client communications in a palliative setting.

There are many times when patients will wish to leave hospice services prematurely. However, hospital internists have been shown to show a significant amount of support for the utilization of hospice services and endorses lengths of stay longer than those currently observed (Iwashyna & Christakis, 1999, p. 241). Anger might also arise from personal fears of hospice patients. Patients express varying levels of trust in regards to healthcare, which range from complete trust to total mistrust. These attitudes have also been found to affect patient outlooks on euthanasia. Also, patients who anticipate fear of meaningless suffering along with lack of belief in hospice services are more likely to advocate euthanasia (Karlsson, 2011, p. 5). Once again, a patient-centered, normative, and empathetic outlook will work to ease the concerns of angry patients and once again establish healthy lines of communication and positive outlooks toward hospice services.

Patient-client communicative relationships should also be virtual, mutual, and ethical in nature. Mutuality in an ethical relationship is founded on the basis of Aristotelian notion of virtuous friendship. Relationship should be built on the principles of reversibility (roles are interchangeable), non-sustainability (personas are irreplaceable apart from their roles), and similitude (an exchange between solicitude and self-esteem) (Olthuis, 2007, p. 78).

Opposing Viewpoints

Sometimes hospice staff will face dilemmas of either adhering to professional care standards or to the wishes of the patients and their families. Hospice care professionals should correctly act according to a set of proper ethical codes, to institutional mission statements, and to professional care standards. However, due to the subjective nature of interpreting such codes, concern and questions of care, as well as conflicts, may arise among the patients themselves, family member, nurses, and doctors (Walker & Breitsameter, 2012, p. 1).

As previously stated, treatment options can be highly influenced by cultural contexts. Iranmanesh, Rayyani, and Forouzy (2012) found that Iranian palliative care nurses showed no tendency to accept the family of patients of the patients themselves as decision makers or to involve them in treatment (p. 9). While I am strongly objected to a viewpoint of healthcare which does not consider the input of the patients themselves, I realize that such a viewpoint may hold as logical in certain cultural contexts. However, regardless of cultural values, the main reason I disagree with such a view point is because it has been scientifically proven that patient satisfaction within a palliative setting is purely subjective (Tierney, Horton, Hannan, & Tierney, 1998, p. 333).

Oduncu and Sahm (2010) found that physicians must make difficult decisions regarding end-of-life care (p. 371). This was no doubt the case for Dr. Daniel Matlock who had an issue with a patient at the University of Colorado Hospital. The woman, in her 70s, became unresponsive after a stroke. The woman had been put on a ventilator by the ambulance crew and then on intravenous fluids by the attending physician. However, she had drafted an advance directive which clearly stated that no life support or artificial nutrition should be given. Therefore, Dr. Matlock consulted the patient's power of attorney, her sister, and then suggested the stopping of the IV. A few days later, the woman was transferred to the hospital's hospice unit where the IV was removed and she passed away. However, Dr. Matlock's colleague was so upset that he referred to Dr. Matlock as a criminal and a Nazi.

In retrospect, I believe Dr. Matlock had taken the correct course of action. Not only did he respect the patient's affirmed wishes, but he also gave the woman a gentler death. It is common knowledge within palliative care that the administering of fluid to dying patients increases secretion and makes breathing even more difficult (Span 2012). This was only one of many cases where respecting the personal wishes of hospice patients and their family members have led to a more beneficial outcome.

Conclusion

In conclusion, a normative and culturally-sensitive attitude should be adopted by health professionals toward hospice and palliative care. It has been proven that a normative approach within a clinical environment as it provides the greatest subjective positive health outcomes of the patient. Also, a culturally-sensitive approach in regards to health care provides optimal health benefits as it considers barriers to patient care which may arise due to the individual characteristics of the patients. Open, ethical, and mutual lines of communication between healthcare professionals and patients should also be stressed as they have been proven to decrease patient frustration and increase patient quality of life. In the end, the old adage that the patient is always right holds firm and palliative care is no different. As health professionals, we must always consider and highly value the input of patients and their families.

6

References

Barnett, L. R. N. (1991). Hospice nurses' knowledge and attitudes toward the near-death experience. *Journal of Near-Death Studies, 9*(4), 225-232.

Barrocas, A., Geppert, C., Durfee, S. M., Maillet, J. O. S., Monturo, C., Mueller, C., ... & Valentine, C. (2010). ASPEN ethics position paper. *Nutrition in Clinical Practice, 25*(6), 672-679.

Blair, L. (1995). Habits of death. Cultural variation in attitudes toward death. *Canadian Family Physician, 41*, 515.

Casarett, D. J., & Quill, T. E. (2007). "I'm not ready for hospice": Strategies for timely and effective hospice discussions. *Annals of Internal Medicine, 146*(6), 443-449.

Casarett, D., Karlawish, J., Morales, K., Crowley, R., Mirsch, T., & Asch, D. A. (2005). Improving the use of hospice services in nursing homes. *JAMA: the journal of the American Medical Association, 294*(2), 211-217.

Catlin, A., Volat, D., Hadley, M. A., Bassir, R., Armigo, C., Valle, E., ... & Anderson, K. (2008). Conscientious objection: a potential neonatal nursing response to care orders that cause suffering at the end of life? Study of a concept. *Neonatal Network: The Journal of Neonatal Nursing, 27*(2), 101-108.

Daniels, N. (2001). Is there a right to health-care, and, if so, what does it encompass?. In H.

Kuhse & P. Singer (Eds.), *A Companion to Bioethics* (pp. 316-325). Oxford: Blacwell Publishing Ltd.

Enguidanos, S., Kogan, A. C., Lorenz, K., & Taylor, G. (2011). Use of role model stories to overcome barriers to hospice among African Americans. *Journal of Palliative Medicine, 14*(2), 161-168.

Goldman, A. I. (1979). What is justified belief?. In *Justification and knowledge* (pp. 1-23). Springer Netherlands.

Houston, R. E. (1999). The angry dying patient. *Primary care companion to the Journal of clinical psychiatry, 1*(1), 5.

Iranmanesh, S., Rayyani, M., & Forouzy, M.A. (2012). Caring at the end of life: Iranian nurses' view and experiences. *Journal of Nursing Education and Practice, 2*(2), p9.

Iwashyna, T. J., & Christakis, N. A. (1998). Attitude and self-reported practice regarding hospice referral in a national sample of internists. *Journal of palliative medicine, 1*(3), 241-248.

Johnson, K. S., Kuchibhatla, M., & Tulsky, J. A. (2008). What explains racial differences in the use of advance directives and attitudes toward hospice care?. *Journal of the American Geriatrics Society, 56*(10), 1953-1958.

Karlsson, M. (2011). *End-of-life care and euthanasia: attitudes of medical students and dying cancer patients.* Inst för onkologi-patologi/Dept of Oncology-Pathology.

Levinson, W., Lesser, C. S., & Epstein, R. M. (2010). Developing physician communication skills for patient-centered care. *Health Affairs, 29*(7), 1310-1318.

Miller, S. C., & Mor, V. N. (2002). The role of hospice care in the nursing home setting. *Journal of palliative medicine, 5*(2), 271-277.

Oduncu, F., & Sahm, S. "Doctor-cared dying instead of physician-assisted suicide: a perspective from Germany." *Medicine, Health Care and Philosophy* 13.4 (2010): 371-381.

Olthuis, G. J. (2007). *Who cares? An ethical study of the moral attitude of professionals in palliative care practice.* [Sl: sn].

Olthuis, G., Leget, C., & Dekkers, W. (2007). Why hospice nurses need high self-esteem. *Nursing ethics, 14*(1), 62-71.

Rainey, L. C., Crane, L. A., Breslow, D. M., & Ganz, P. A. (1984). Cancer patients' attitudes toward hospice services. *CA: a cancer journal for clinicians, 34*(4), 191-201.

Seamark, D. A., Thorne, C. P., Jones, R. V., Gray, D. J., & Searle, J. F. (1993). Knowledge and perceptions of a domiciliary hospice service among general practitioners and community nurses. *The British Journal of General Practice, 43*(367), 57.

Span, Paula. "Among Doctors, Fierce Reluctance to Let Go." *The New Old Age Among Doctors Fierce Reluctance to Let Go Comments.* The New York Times, 29 Mar. 2012. Web. 16 Nov. 2013. <http://newoldage.blogs.nytimes.com/2012/03/29/among-doctors-fierce-reluctance-to-let-go/?_r=0>.

Tierney, R. M., Horton, S. M., Hannan, T. J., & Tierney, W. M. (1998). Relationships between symptom relief, quality of life, and satisfaction with hospice care. *Palliative Medicine, 12*(5), 333-344.

Walker, A., & Breitsameter, C. (2012). Conflicts and conflict regulation in hospices: nurses' perspectives. *Medicine, Health Care and Philosophy*, 1-10.